Apple Cider Vinegar

The Ultimate Guide to Losing Weight and Feeling Amazing with One Food!

By: Natalie Ray

Disclaimer

The author of this book is not affiliated with any medical company, nor does the author provide medical treatment advice in any way. The ideas, views, and opinions expressed in this book are those of the author. The author assumes no liability for advice or suggestions offered in this book. The author and publisher of this book and the accompanying materials have used their best efforts in preparing this book. The author and publisher make no representation or warranties with respect to the accuracy, applicability, fitness, or completeness of the contents of this book. The information contained in this book is strictly for informational purposes. Therefore, if you wish to apply ideas contained in this book, you are taking full responsibility for your actions.

Table of Contents

Introduction

Some of the most basic products that sit in our pantry are also the most ignored. Instead of going back to what our forefathers used to battle ailments and stay healthy, as a society we tend to turn to prescriptions and medications these days. While some prescriptions are certainly needed in a person's life to help with a condition, there are also instances where a natural remedy might do the trick a bit better.

What ingredient could this possibly be? Apple cider vinegar. This age old item is probably sitting in a plastic container at the back of your pantry collecting dust right now. When was the last time you cooked with it? When was the last time you did anything with it besides move it around on the shelf? Chances are it has been a long time. Probably too long if you are a person who suffers from one or many different chronic conditions or ailments that you would like to fix.

Apple cider has so many positive benefits when you use it that it requires an entire eBook to discuss them. There are uses around the house, with the pets and a ton of them when it comes to the human body. There are benefits to a person's skin, weight, breathing, metabolism, oral care and organ health when just a little bit of vinegar is used occasionally. Imagine how healthy a person can be when the apple cider vinegar is used on a regular basis? There is even a chance you could get rid of some of the prescriptions sitting in your bathroom with just a little bit of cider vinegar added to your daily routine.

Losing weight is a great way to get healthy and very easy to do if you choose to follow the apple cider vinegar diet. By losing weight with the apple cider vinegar diet you will have more energy, feel better about yourself and look great in clothes that used to fit (a few sizes ago). Dropping a few pounds is also a great way to improve your health since extra weight increases your risk for cancer, diabetes, heart disease, stroke and many other chronic ailments.

Apple cider vinegar is safe for the body. After all, it is an all natural ingredient found in nature. It isn't a prescription pill and it doesn't have any harmful side effects. Apple cider vinegar is simply a product from nature that works within the body to quickly and efficiently burn off calories, fend off diseases and work with the body's chemistry to produce many good results.

Chapter 1 – What is Apple Cider Vinegar?

Apple cider vinegar is something that has been around for hundreds of years. It was readily available for your ancestors because it is simply made from apples. That's it. The apples are pressed and the juice and even bits of apples are allowed to sit and ferment for months at a time until vinegar has formed.

Apple cider vinegar is also known as cider vinegar. It can be purchased from the store and comes in regular, organic and unpasteurized forms. There are different forms of vinegar made because people have a lot of uses for the vinegar ranging from using it in a household cleaner to using it as an ingredient in a salad dressing.

Cider vinegar can also be made in the home with just a few tools and some apples. Once you become a believer in what apple cider vinegar can do for your own health and that of your family's, you might want to consider making it in your own home. It is a little bit cheaper and you can make it in a large volume, as long as you have the place to store it while it ferments.

Why should you care about apple cider vinegar? Because it is like a super hero when it comes to ingredients that can be used to better a person's health. There are so many ways that apple cider is beneficial to a human that it takes several chapters just to cover them all. Since you are reading this eBook that means you are interested in adding apple cider vinegar to your diet and maybe even your beauty routine.

But just in case you become hooked, here is one of the easiest recipes to follow to make your own apple cider vinegar at home. The recipe can be doubled or tripled depending on the space you have to process the apples and let it sit and ferment.

Making Apple Cider Vinegar

Making the cider is a very simple process. Once the apples are pressed and you have it sitting around and fermenting, that's about all you need to worry about. Check the bowl or jars frequently and monitor how it is coming occasionally, but that is it.

Ingredients:

Apples (fall or winter variety)
Jars
Cheesecloth

There isn't a set amount for how many apples to use with this recipe. You can use a small amount if you are living alone or you can process a large amount, if you have a large family and household to maintain. The only thing you do need to have is jars to handle the liquid that is pressed from the amount of apples you choose.

Wash the apples and then crush them so you can retain the juice. It is OK if apple pulp gets in the liquid as it can be filtered off at a later time.

Pour the liquid in to cleaned jars or large bowls. Do not fill them completely full. Store the juice in a room where they will not receive direct sunlight and where the temperature can be controlled. A dark room that is climate controlled is the best option if you have it. Cover the jars or the bowls with cheesecloth or loosely with a lid.

If you are in more of a hurry to have vinegar at your disposal, there is a type of yeast that will speed up the fermentation process. This is not the same kind of yeast you use to prepare bread or rolls. This yeast is specific to liquids and the same as what is used in the alcohol making process. The grocery store might carry this product or you can check with the local wine retailer if they sell homebrew supplies. Crumble the blocks of yeast up according to the package directions. The yeast will usually cut the fermentation time in half versus if you were to let it sit on its own.

Each day, stir the contents of the jar and replace the covering whether you use the yeast or not. This process will take at least 4 weeks of stirring before the vinegar is at the level where you want it to be without yeast. With yeast it will take approximately two to three weeks. For stronger vinegars, you can opt to let it sit and ferment longer.

When the vinegar is at the fermentation level you desire, it needs to be strained. Pour it through a coffee filter or several layers of cheesecloth in to a cleaned and sterile jar. Place a lid securely over the vinegar and it is ready for use.

Vinegar will not spoil and it will last a long time if it is stored in a cool location out of sunlight – like in the pantry. Make several bottles and keep them in various places around the house so they are convenient to grab when you need some vinegar to perform a task. The vinegar can be diluted and placed in spray bottles right away in rooms where you will be cleaning, such as the bathrooms and the laundry room.

The Popularity of Apple Cider Vinegar

Apple cider was used to clean the house, it was used to treat just about every skin ailment under the sun and it worked on a host of other problems as well. It was a very common item in every house for the last couple of hundred years. Then modern medicine hit the scene and old world remedies like apple cider vinegar were forgotten and replaced with medicines that were surely more effective.

The health benefits were just shrugged off and only a small percentage of people continued to use the vinegar until it was virtually forgotten about in the highly advanced and technological world we live in. But just like with anything else in the world, it doesn't really catch on or become a trend until a celebrity or two talks about how they have experienced the benefits of a product. The same is true for apple cider vinegar's health benefits and the diet that is related to it. (See chapter 3 to learn about the diet specifically). There were people who followed the principles of the diet, but until models and actresses began talking about it, it was considered one of those things that "health nuts" did. Now it has become popular again to use the all natural method to clean the house and take advantage of natural remedies that can solve medical issues.

No longer is apple cider vinegar something that only health nuts do. Sure, the people who use it as a regular part of their day care about their health and want to improve it, but they are not nuts. They are very smart and well educated on knowing how to take care of their bodies so they can last a long time. The use of apple cider vinegar will only increase in the future as the majority of the population ages and people want to combat the effects of their age.

Caution: While taking apple cider vinegar daily as a part of a person' diet has shown many healthful benefits, there are a few cautions to be aware of. First, vinegar is highly acidic and consuming it regularly could irritate the throat. Secondly, apple cider could contain properties that when consumed in too large of an amount it may cause gastric distress and diarrhea. Only consume it in the recommended doses to stay healthy.

Chapter 2 – Improve Your Health

Adding apple cider vinegar to your diet on a regular basis helps your health in many ways. One of the most important ways is that it makes the blood balanced in terms of its pH level. Even though apple cider vinegar contains acetic acid, once it is digested in the body it raises the chemical balance to be a higher alkaline level. Why is this important?

A body that has an acidic balance is prone to diseases and infections. An acidic environment allows bad cells, such as cancer cells, to develop rapidly throughout the body. When the body has an alkaline balance, the bad cells are kept in check and even prevented from multiplying and causing issues within the body. Since apple cider vinegar makes the body lean more towards an alkaline chemical makeup, it is a great thing to have in the diet. The more regularly you consume the apple cider vinegar, the longer the body will remain at an alkaline level.

Another important reason to ingest apple cider vinegar on a regular basis is because it helps to flush out the blood and the body's cells. When a person has a diet high in salt, they will retain water; look and feel bloated and hold in toxins that need to be flushed out. By drinking or eating a moderate amount of apple cider vinegar, those toxins and the salt are flushed out faster because of the properties it contains. This doesn't mean you should drink straight cider vinegar in a large amount, it simply means that by diluting it with water or adding it to another beverage it can help get the bad stuff out faster. The faster the bad stuff is out, the better you will feel.

Besides those major accomplishments that vinegar can do in your body, it is also responsible for a whole lot more. By adding just a bit of apple cider vinegar to your diet you can see a whole host of problems disappear in just a matter of a few days. Some of the benefits that are known but not necessarily felt may include:

- Naturally balanced sugar levels. Apple cider vinegar regulates the sugar in the blood and keeps it at even levels which could also stave off diabetes from developing. A balanced sugar level will keep a person from experiencing spikes in energy and lulls from downtime.

- Decreased bloating. The properties in vinegar work to eliminate the foods that cause bloating – fatty, greasy foods – faster so they do not stick around and cause you to look and feel bloated.

- Increased circulation. The blood that is clean and flowing through your system after a dose of apple cider vinegar circulates better than blood that is full of chemicals from food, prescription drugs and even other additives from a diet.

Even though apple cider vinegar is responsible for curing many ailments in the body, it is probably most popular because of how it helps the body to lose weight. Once it was discovered by people – researchers as well as actresses and models who wanted to stay thin – it became a widely talked about substance that was a must have for any dieter.

Chapter 3 –Lose Weight by Consuming Apple Cider Vinegar

A person can take apple cider vinegar throughout the day and not be on the apple cider vinegar diet. Some people only take a small amount each day, such as a teaspoon mixed in their morning tea or as an ingredient in their salad dressing. Other people who want to be healthy but also drop an amount of weight will consume it in a slightly higher dose. Consuming it in a higher dose can be done once a day by drinking a diluted beverage or it can be interspersed all day long by including certain recipes in the diet.

Even though cider vinegar has shown dramatic results in regards to weight loss, it isn't a substitution for eating healthy and exercising. For example, it isn't a smart idea to eat eggs, bacon and donuts for breakfast each day and claim that you are healthy because you add a teaspoon of vinegar to the coffee each morning. Being healthy is a round the clock adventure which you should always be striving for. You can have an occasional donut or bacon, but do it sparingly and eat a high protein low fat breakfast that is better for you the majority of the time.

If you are a person who has a healthy diet overall and want to get your daily dose of vinegar out of the way at one time, then consider taking it as a drink. For every 16 ounces of water you have, add 2 teaspoons of the vinegar and mix it well. You don't need to add vinegar to the water all day long, just once in the day is probably adequate. Too much could cause you to have diarrhea.

How the Diet Works

There are a lot of ways in which the apple cider vinegar helps the body to shed pounds when you are following the diet. The vinegar helps to flush the bloodstream of toxins, it helps to suppress the appetite, it boosts the metabolism and it breaks down the fat faster. No wonder why there are such good results seen after having just apple cider vinegar for just a few weeks.

Suppresses the Appetite

Apples are loaded with vitamin B and pectin, which give the body energy and help to make the stomach feel full. The cider vinegar is obviously made from apples, so it contains those same properties that make the body feel full. Some researchers and dieticians have suggested that a person who is really trying to lose a lot of weight should do is take one teaspoon of vinegar thirty minutes before each meal. They can opt to drink it plain or mix with water, tea or juice. Giving it thirty minutes to settle will allow you time to feel full before you sit down and eat a plate laden with food.

Boosts the Energy

Vitamin B is one ingredient that is all the rage right now. It is what is extracted and put in to energy drinks in order to give a person energy. By eating an apple or having some cider vinegar instead of an energy drink, you can get just as much energy without all of the harmful chemicals and additives put in with it. Everybody knows that the more energy you have, the more you move around. The more you move around, the more calories you burn.

Increased Levels of Metabolism

By adding the acid to your stomach via the form of vinegar, you are setting yourself up to breakdown the food entering it at a much faster rate. Acids contained in the vinegar bust up fat and process the food bits much faster than if you didn't have the cider beforehand. The faster the food is processed, the higher your metabolism will be. The more you can metabolize at a higher rate, the faster the excess pounds will be burned off.

Process the Fat Out

A body that metabolizes fast means that it doesn't allow food to sit around and take up space – such as in a spare tire, on the hips, on the thighs or any other unwanted place on the body. Since the body is metabolizing quickly the fat doesn't get the chance to deposit inside and is simply processed out right away. The faster the fat processes, the faster your body can get to burning off the stored fat on your frame. Burning stored fat is done when you exercise to burn it off.

Control the Sugar Cravings

The natural acids in the cider vinegar also help block cravings, especially those for sugary products. Sugar is full of empty calories and not good for the body. The less sugar laden foods one consumes, the less time they have to waste burning off sugar calories. They can go right to burning off the stored fat when they work out instead of having to start over each time and use up the sugar calories before it can process on to the fat calories.

In short, the apple cider vinegar diet can work in one of several ways. You need to choose the method that works the best for you and what fits in to your lifestyle, not what other experts necessarily recommend.

Method A – consume 1 tsp of apple cider vinegar before each meal. Build up to 1 tbsp to suppress the appetite.

Method B – Add apple cider vinegar in to your meals and follow a healthy diet and incorporate exercise in to your daily routine.

Method C – Eat your normal healthy diet and drink apple cider vinegar diluted in water each day.

The right answer might also be a combination of the above ideas. The best thing about working with the apple cider vinegar diet is that there are no hard and fast rules that have to be followed, making its flexibility very easy for those who do choose to use it.

Chapter 4 – Recipes with Apple Cider Vinegar

Coming up with recipes to follow within the guidelines of the apple cider vinegar are a little bit tricky because it isn't an ingredient that can just be added to any dish. For example, would you put a dash of vinegar over your baked potato or dessert? Probably not. There are ways you can incorporate it in to certain dishes so that you don't even know you are eating or drinking it.

Depending on how strictly you are going to follow the diet rules will determine how much you need to consume each day. But remember, too much of a good thing can also be bad for you as well. Stick within the guidelines for how much vinegar is recommended throughout the day in order to avoid getting sick.

The best way to use cider vinegar is in sauces or dressings and put over top of healthy entrees and side dishes you are preparing. Some enthusiasts who use apple cider vinegar claim that it can be used in place of lemon in any recipe you use. However, check the recipe carefully as the vinegar might be a bit overpowering where the lemon was supposed to be. You could also try using a smaller amount to see if the taste didn't interfere and then gradually add more if the taste wasn't too powerful.

For other dishes, you can come up with some tasty meals using apple cider vinegar so you don't have to drink a teaspoon or a tablespoon of it plain before a meal. Vinegar is one basic ingredient to marinades for any type of meat and also in dressings, so use it!

Breakfast

Getting apple cider in to your diet in the early morning hours might be a challenge. Sprinkling it over scrambled eggs or toast just doesn't seem feasible, so you will probably need to rely on a beverage to get the day started off right.

Apple & Honey Water

Not quite apple juice, not quite apple cider. Something even better than the two!

2 tsp apple cider vinegar
1 tbsp honey
1-2 cups water

Pour all of the ingredients in to a mug and heat in the microwave until hot. Stir with a cinnamon stick and serve warm.

Fruity Juice

With so many fruits mixed in this drink, you won't know it is healthy for you.

Ingredients:

½ cup cider vinegar

2 cups water

1 tsp lemon juice

½ cup grape juice

1 tsp honey

½ tsp cinnamon

Measure all of the ingredients in to a large pitcher. If you have a really big one, you can double the recipe so that you don't have to make it as often. Refrigerate until you are ready to serve with breakfast or pour over ice and enjoy at any time of the day.

Lunch & Dinner

The easiest method to getting cider vinegar in to your diet is by adding it to a recipe for salad dressing. Since the best dressings are vinaigrettes anyway, it isn't a stretch to include the apple cider vinegar as one of the main ingredients for it. But don't count out the meats and the side dishes quite yet. Following are several dressing recipes that will also work as a marinade for chicken, pork and lean beef.

Berry Salad with Dressing

This salad is especially delicious during the summer months when you can use fresh greens and berries.

Ingredients:
1 cup spinach leaves
1 cup sliced strawberries
1 cup blueberries
1 cup olive oil
2/3 cup apple cider vinegar
¼ cup sugar

In a large bowl, combine the washed spinach leaves with the washed and prepared fruit.

In a small bowl, mix the oil, vinegar and sugar until it is combined. Drizzle over the salad and eat right away.

Basic Vinaigrette Dressing

The basic vinaigrette dressing is commonly used on salads, but it can also be drizzled over a baked potato, on vegetables and used to dip breadsticks in.

<u>Ingredients:</u>
1 cup cider vinegar
2 tbsp mustard
1/2 tbsp curry
1/2 cup chopped chives
1/3 cup lemon juice
3/4 cup virgin olive oil

In a bowl, whisk together the vinegar, mustard, curry and chives until they are blended. Add the olive oil in and continue to whisk until they ingredients are all mixed. Pour over salad o other food and eat accordingly.

Honey & Vinegar

This recipe is great over a salad loaded with veggies, but it also takes the place of honey mustard dressing which can be full of extra calories you don't need.

Ingredients:

2 tbsp olive oil
1 clove crushed garlic
3 tbsp apple cider vinegar
3 tbsp plain yogurt – fat free
¼ tsp honey

Place all of the ingredients in an emulsifier or a blender if you have one. Shake them rapidly until they are well mixed. Drizzle over salad greens and then serve cold.

Garlic Oil

This recipe is good to serve over a salad, but it is even better when you drizzle it over roasted or grilled vegetables. Vegetables such as carrots, summer squash, onions and peppers make for a great combination to slice up and roast on a cookie sheet in the oven or in the grill pan over medium heat.

<u>Ingredients:</u>
3 tbsp canola oil
3 tbsp apple cider vinegar
1 crushed garlic clove
Salt and pepper

In a small dish or a blender, combine all of the ingredients until they are well mixed.
Immediately sprinkle over vegetables and place in the oven or drizzle over a fresh salad.

Garlic Chicken

Chicken is one of the leanest meats there is, so use it often and with apple cider vinegar when you are able. This recipe is simple and delicious.

<u>Ingredients:</u>
6 skinless, boneless chicken breasts
5 teaspoons garlic salt
1 cup cider vinegar

Grease a 9 x 13 pan. Sprinkle the salt over the breasts and then drizzle the oil on top of the salt. Bake at 350 degrees for 30 to 40 minutes or until juices run out clear.

Veggie Salad

Having a garden in the backyard will produce a lot of vegetables that you get to eat as soon as they are ripe. Utilize those veggies in this salad that also calls for rice.

Ingredients:
2 cups cooked brown rice
3 tbsp cider vinegar
2 tbsp olive oil
2 tbsp parsley
½ tsp sugar
1 cup cherry tomatoes – diced
½ cup celery – diced
1/3 cup onion – diced

In a large bowl, add all of the prepared vegetables.

In a separate bowl, mix the vinegar, oil, parsley and sugar with a whisk. Drizzle over the vegetables and then toss until they are all coated.

Serve over the prepared rice.

Crockpot Pork Roast

When you have a busy family, it is important to have dishes that you can throw in a slow roaster in the morning and come home to find they are done!

<u>Ingredients:</u>
One three to five pound pork roast
1 tbsp vegetable oil
1 cup apple cider vinegar
1 ½ cup ketchup
½ cup molasses
1/3 cup mustard
2 cloves of minced garlic
2 tsp pepper
2 tsp cumin
2 tsp coriander
2 tsp paprika
2 tsp cornstarch
1 tbsp chili pepper
½ tsp salt

In a small bowl, mix the oil, chili powder, pepper, cumin, coriander, paprika, salt and garlic in to a paste. Rub it thoroughly over the roast and place in the bottom of the crock pot. Allow to sit on low for at least one hour.

In another bowl, mix the vinegar, molasses and mustard. Pour it over the roast and then turn on to the low setting for 8 hours or until the meat is tender.

Meatballs

These meatballs are delicious because they are baked in the oven and make little mess compared to frying them in a pan. Toss them in a crock pot or a baking dish and add the sauce to make them even yummier.

Ingredients:
1 can crushed pineapple
1/2 cup apple cider vinegar
1/4 cup brown sugar
2 tbsp soy sauce
1 teaspoon ginger
1 1/2 pounds lean ground beef
3/4 cup bread crumbs
1/4 cup skim milk
1/2 tsp salt
1 tbsp canola oil
1 tbsp water
1 tbsp cornstarch
1 egg

Drain the pineapple and reserve the liquid in to a small bowl. Add the water to the juice until there is ¾ of a cup full of liquid. Add the vinegar, soy sauce, brown sugar and ginger.

In another bowl, mix the ground beef and the remaining ingredients by hand until they are well blended. Form in to balls and place on a baking sheet. Bake at 350 degrees for 3o minutes or until juices run clear.

In the bottom of the Crockpot, transfer the meatballs. Pour the juice over the top and cook on low for two hours. Add the cornstarch and the water and cook for an additional 4 to six hours on low.

Stone Soup

OK, so there's really not a stone in the soup but that would be a fun story. This recipe has lots of great vegetables and the cider to keep you healthy.

<u>Ingredients:</u>
2 carrots – diced
2 parsnips – peeled and chopped
1 sweet potato, cubed
1 beet, peeled and cube
1 onion, diced
½ cup cider vinegar
1 tbsp olive oil
8 cups water
Salt and pepper to taste

In a large stock pot, sauté the onions with the oil until they are soft. Add the remaining vegetables on group at a time and cook for five minutes before adding the next group. Pour the water over the top and reduce the heat to low and allow to simmer for at least two hours or until the vegetables are to the desired tenderness. Add the vinegar and heat through before serving.

Snacks

Healthy snacks are needed to keep your energy level up through the day. Apple cider vinegar can be added to several dishes if you need to get a bit more in for the day. The vinegar can be added in to a dip or a sauce that you use with fruits or vegetables when you need to grab a snack on the run or if you are just chilling out at home.

Olive Oil

There are times when you just need to have a bit of carbs to get you through a day. Instead of loading down a piece of fresh French bread with butter, opt for an olive oil dip.

<u>Ingredients:</u>
3 tbsp olive oil
3 tbsp apple cider vinegar
Salt

Add all three ingredients in to a shaker container. Mix until they are well combined and spread out on to a plate with a lip. Dip chunks of fresh French baguette pieces.

Chapter 5 – Beauty Tips Using Apple Cider Vinegar

Even though all of the ways in which cider vinegar can help you lose weight are impressive, the most interesting reasons to use it haven't been discussed. Sure, the vinegar will help you to drop pounds, but it can also help your skin, hair and nails to look and stay beautiful.

Skin

Cider vinegar helps the skin in several different ways. If you thought you were going to live the rest of your life with imperfect skin, think again. Apple cider vinegar is better than any $1,000 per ounce cream or concealer on the market. It is so versatile that you could have incredible skin just by using this product.

This is just a few of the best ways in which apple cider vinegar improves the skin:

Conceals a host of Imperfections

- Cider vinegar can be rubbed over the facial skin, hands, feet or any area that contains age spots. The spots will gradually lighten until they are almost invisible in just a matter of weeks.

- Rub the cider vinegar over any varicose veins that appear on the legs or even veins that start to show on the face. The vinegar's shrinking properties will make them appear smaller and not bump out or show through the skin like they normally do. The inflammation will also be reduced if they are painful and bulging because of the pressure on them when you stand.

- The apple cider vinegar can be applied to the face or back region where acne breakouts have occurred. The vinegar will lessen the scars and hide the redness if there as any that is associated with current breakouts.

- Using a rinse of apple cider vinegar on your hair after shampooing will help moisturize the scalp and lessen the case of dandruff. The scalp will no longer be itchy or have flakes.

- For people who suffer from psoriasis, applying cider vinegar over inflamed areas will reduce the inflammation and the redness. Continued use of the vinegar over the skin will also help prevent future outbreaks.

- The skin can get tired after being shaved every single day. Mix a concoction of half water and half cider vinegar and use as an aftershave to cool hot and irritated skin.

- Using warm water and vinegar wash your face with a soft cloth. The cider vinegar will help to remove blackheads and keep pimples from appearing on the skin.

- Every woman hates to see cellulite on her body. Rubbing apple cider vinegar over the troubled spots will helps to soften the bumps and to make the skin appear smoother around the desired region.

Hair

Cider vinegar makes average looking hair gorgeous after a few uses. The properties of the vinegar strip away the residue and the chemicals that build up after frequent washing. To get great looking hair, simply shampoo like normal but rinse with the apple cider vinegar. As mentioned above, it helps reduce dandruff but it will also make your hair shiny and glossy, just like in the magazine pictures.

For the men, they can also rinse with cider vinegar after shampooing but they need to take it a step farther. They need to massage their scalp with the vinegar. The cider will stimulate the hair follicles and it encourages hair to grow back. A full head of hair might not grow, but it could prevent premature baling or a bald spot from appearing.

Nails

Since apples are loaded with naturally occurring pectin it is no wonder that cider vinegar helps them too. Pectin is the naturally occurring ingredient that makes nails strong. The more frequently you consume apple cider vinegar, the stronger the nails will be. They will not be as dry not crack or chip as easily.

For the people who have sensitive skin, they may want to try diluting the apple cider vinegar with water before they put it on any part of their skin. Chances are the cider will do no harm, however it is better to be cautious on the first use and make sure rather than have a skin irritation develop. After the initial trial and there are no problems, then go ahead and use straight vinegar on the skin to get all of its healing potential.

Chapter 6 – Curing Other Ailments

Cider vinegar helps a person lose weight, balances their blood sugar, improves many skin conditions, helps the hair and nails to grow and wards off chronic disease. Can you believe there are still a whole host of other ailments that apple cider vinegar combats too?

<u>Lowers Cholesterol</u>

The proteins in the vinegar are helpful to break down the fat that is consumed at meal time. The vinegar can also get in to the blood stream and clean out the fatty deposits known as cholesterol. A cholesterol buildup in the veins can lead to stroke or heart disease, both of which can be fatal if not controlled. Therefore, start a diet of regular apple cider vinegar consumption and the cholesterol can be reduced significantly without the aid of prescriptions. If your doctor has you on a prescription, continue taking it but if your levels are lowered enough, they might be able to remove you from the medicine.

Bioscience, Biotechnology and Biochemistry published a report in 2009 that said the people in their study who consumed the acetic acid from the cider vinegar for three months had a significantly lower body weight, triglyceride level, abdominal fat and waist circumference. All of those points are big risk indicators for a heart attack, so whenever there is an easy option to lower them, it is for the betterment of your longevity.

Relieves Insomnia

The properties get in to the blood and do a whole lot of good for the digestion, but it also works well for other systems in the body. The components release materials that relax the body and help it fall asleep and stay asleep during the night. For people who have been insomniacs for months or years, they can be cured simply by drinking a cider tea before bedtime. If they do not like chamomile tea with cider, they could simply opt for water with cider stirred in.

Prevent UTIs

The acid from the vinegar processes through the body in a way that is helpful for the urinary tract. It pushes out toxins and bacteria that can cause infections. Just drinking a little bit a day can keep the kidneys and the bladder clear from bacteria.

Eliminate Candida

Candida is yeast cells that grow naturally in the body when it has an excess of sugar. The more sugar, the more Candida there will be. Candida can cause yeast infections, disrupt the sleep and cause poor performance during work or school hours. By drinking or eating vinegar cider, the Candida fail to thrive and grow, thereby reducing the symptoms or eliminating them completely.

Sunburns

Sunburns are very painful to live with, especially when they happen in sensitive areas. However, a bit of apple cider vinegar applied shortly after you realize you are burned can immediately provide relief. Apply the cider vinegar to a paper towel or a thin cloth. For severe burns, make sure the cloth is soaked. Place the soaked towel over the skin and allow it to sit for ten minutes. Reapply the cider vinegar and then move the cloth around to another affected area. Repeat this process until all of the affected areas have been covered.

This process can be repeated continuously without any ill effects other than being stinky. Applying the cider vinegar to the skin will take the heat out of it immediately. The longer you keep the skin moist with vinegar, the less chance there is that it will peel once it begins to heal as well. With several applications in the evening hours, the pinkness might be completely gone by the next morning since it works so well.

Removes Warts

A wart is another skin issue that vinegar takes care of. Dab a cotton ball in to the vinegar and place it over the wart. You can cover the cotton ball with tape or a band aid to hold on securely for several hours or you can apply it several times throughout the day for one week. After one week the wart should flake off and leave no marks or scars.

Reduces Foot Swelling

Standing on your feet all day can cause them to swell. Heat, pregnancy and lack of fluids can also make them swell and ache. To relieve the aches and the swelling, find a bucket or a large pail and add one gallon of water and 1 cup of cider vinegar. The water can be heated or it can remain room temperature. Allow the feet to soak for 20 minutes and the aches and the swelling will disappear.

Oral Care

Your mouth is something you should take very good care of. Anything that forms in the mouth has the possibility to affect the rest of your body, so care for your teeth, gums and all of those taste buds inside. Cider vinegar can help you in several ways when it comes to your oral health.

- Use a soft brush and some water mixed with vinegar. Dip the brush in the mix and softly scrub to clean dentures. The dentures can also be dropped in the cup and allowed to soak overnight so they are disinfected.

- The components within the cider break down bacteria in the mouth that cause bad breath. To fight bad breath, dilute vinegar and water and gargle for 30 seconds. Spit and rinse twice a day to keep the bad breath away.

- Use a toothbrush dipped in vinegar to remove stains on the teeth that are caused from wine, coffee, soda and other dark colored foods. Simply brush the teeth twice a day with the cider and wait for the stains to disappear in one to two weeks.

Fights Allergy Symptoms

People who suffer from seasonal allergies and asthma should take cider vinegar as often as they can during the season when they suffer from allergies the most. The chemical makeup of the vinegar reduces swelling in the nasal passages, but t also blocks excessive mucous production. The snuffling, runny nose and painful pressure can be things of the past just by taking in some vinegar.

Reduces Heartburn

Acid causes heartburn. When the stomach acid builds, it causes the insides of the esophagus to burn. Instead of taking anti-acid pills, drink some apple cider infused water or simply 1 teaspoon of cider straight. Even though it is technically an acid, it digests in the system as a base and will balance out the levels in your stomach.

Prevents Food Poisoning

The acid within the vinegar is also good for your stomach by what it can kill. The acid is strong to foreign objects, such as bacteria that cause food poisoning. The regular stomach enzymes you have aren't threatened by the acid, but ones that aren't supposed to be in your system don't like it.

Chapter 7 – Odds & Ends with Apple Cider Vinegar

There are plenty of healthy benefits to get from using apple cider vinegar. There are also a lot of miscellaneous items that can be done around the house or with your pets so they can both reap some positive results from the ingredient too.

<u>Detoxification</u>

The body naturally stores chemicals it comes in to contact with in the fat cells. Some of these chemicals are from the air that is breathed, from the artificial sweeteners and preservatives that are eaten and even from the prescriptions we take each day. These chemicals build up and can cause a person to be sluggish and carry around extra weight. Apple cider vinegar is an excellent ingredient to use in a cleanse to get rid of those chemicals in a detox.

A detox isn't any lengthy process. It is simply a period of time where you eat raw or pure foods and drink a diluted beverage with apple cider vinegar in it to flush the chemicals out. A detox can rid the body of not only toxins that have been stored up in the cells but also pounds. Those chemicals and toxins can add up in ounces and when they are flushed, you might lose five pounds within a couple of days.

<u>Body</u>

- When you follow a detox plan, the apple cider vinegar cleanses the kidneys at the same time. The cider vinegar runs through the system and as it flushes out the other cells from all of the bad ingredients they are holding, they are pushed out through the kidneys and the excretory system. The cleaner the kidneys are, the more efficient they work at pushing the bad stuff out of the body every day.

- We already know how the cider vinegar can improve the ailments of the skin, but what about injuries? Cider vinegar can be used as a way to soothe jellyfish stings. Simply use a paper towel and dab the vinegar on the sting or else pour the cider right over the top of it. Depending on how much it stings, you can repeat the process as often as possible to soothe the pain.

- Cider vinegar helps nails to grow strong and fast, but it is also used to remove fungus. Apply the cider vinegar with a cotton swab once to twice a day. The fungus will disappear after a few days worth of treatment.

- Besides drinking and eating cider vinegar to draw toxins out of the body, you can bathe in it in order to draw them out of your skin. Fill a bath with warm water and add two to four tablespoons of cider vinegar (depending on how large your tub is). Soak in the vinegar and you will pull the toxins from your skin so is glows when you are done. It can also work to remove any ingrown hairs or slivers while you work at soaking.

- During the summer months when the biting bugs are bad, you or the kids might want to scratch their arms off. Don't! Dilute vinegar with water and apply to the affected area with a paper towel or a damp cloth. The cider vinegar relieves the swelling around a bite and will take away the itching.

By consuming cider vinegar on a regular basis, you are also using it as a preventative measure for your body. The natural ingredients in the apple cider vinegar boost the immune system and enable it to fight against the flu virus in particular. Take your regular amount of cider on a daily basis, but when there is a flu outbreak nearby, think about doubling your intake as an extra barrier from the germs.

There are few things less annoying than having a bad case of the hiccups. Did you know drinking a diluted glass full of water and vinegar will stop the diaphragm from spasms? The spasms are what result in hiccups.

Cleaning Product

Apple cider vinegar is an excellent cleaning product to use around the house. It smells wonderful and it disinfects too!

- Add water and 1 tablespoon of vinegar to a spray bottle that is empty (regular cleaner size). Mist over windows and glass surfaces and wipe with a paper towel. The ingredients will not streak the windows when you clean them.

- To clean the toilets, pour ½ cup of straight vinegar in to the bowl at night, when everyone has used it for the last time. Close the lid and allow the vinegar to sit overnight. Flush it in the morning and it will disinfect and smell good for days.

- To clean appliances, mix water and cider in a two to one ratio. For example, mix 1 cup of cider in a bowl with two cups of water. Dip a sponge or a cloth in the water and then use on the surface or the inside of the refrigerator, the microwave, the dishwasher and the stove. They will also dry with no streaks and no residue.

- If you forgot to buy a new box of detergent, never fear, cider can do the trick. Fill the soap compartment with vinegar and let it run on the normal cleaning cycle.

Pets

The benefits from apple cider vinegar extend out to your furry friends as well! The cider can be used safely with your cat or dog because it is a non-toxic ingredient.

- To keep cats from marking or spraying around the house, use the same spray bottle with diluted vinegar and water and spritz the designated area. If a cat has marked one area, they will return and do it again unless you treat it with vinegar. They do not like the smell of vinegar and will leave it alone.

- Vinegar is also a deterrent to fleas and biting insects that are bothersome to your pet. To prevent them from getting bites and becoming infested, there are two ways you can treat them. The first is to add one teaspoon of vinegar to one gallon of drinking water. They can just drink the water and the vinegar scent that comes out of their pores will deter fleas from staying on their coat. The second method is to bathe them or mist them with the diluted vinegar and water. The only problem is that way doesn't last as long as if they are ingesting the vinegar.

Outdoors

Apple cider vinegar can get rid of bothersome weeds and pests in the yard too. The best part about using apple cider vinegar in the garden and around the house is that it is non-toxic compared to other treatments used to kill weeds and pests. This means it is safe for the children to play outside as soon as you apply a treatment around the yard. It also means that your pets don't have to stay locked up indoors while the grass dries and becomes less toxic for them.

- To kill weeds that have grown up through the cracks in the sidewalk, the divider in the drive way or in the landscaping, pour the cider vinegar directly over it. Make sure the leaves are completely coated with the vinegar and in a matter of days the weeds will wilt and die completely. You can then pull them out of the ground easily and throw them away. Straight form kills weeds
- Pests such as aphids can easily be killed with one application of cider vinegar treatment. Mix a solution that contains one gallon of water and 2 tablespoons of cider together and put in a watering can or a large spray bottle. Spray over the infested area twice a day or until there are no more aphids or bugs hanging out and destroying your plants.

Conclusion

Is your head spinning from all of the benefits there are just from adding one simple ingredient in your life? Now, the question is how much apple cider vinegar should you buy to stock the pantry instead of just wondering how long it has been sitting in the same spot? Between the plans you have made to include it in your diet, now you have to consider how many changes you will make in your beauty routine and when you will have a chance to clean around the house and smell the results for yourself.

Use cider vinegar in as many places as you can manage in order to garner the most results. Think not only of the healthy benefits that your body gets from consuming cider vinegar, but from the lack of other ingredients being put in to your body. The more apple cider vinegar you use as a cleaning agent around the house, the less chemicals there will be floating around the air for you to inhale. The fewer toxins there are to inhale, the less free radicals there are to bounce around and produce cancer cells in your body.

Apple cider vinegar is a fairly inexpensive item that can do wonders for your body. Give it a try and once you see the results for yourself, you will be hooked on it and trying to get your friends and family to use apple cider vinegar too.